# Nourishing Recipes For A Healthy Gallbladder:

## Delicious Meals for Optimal Digestion

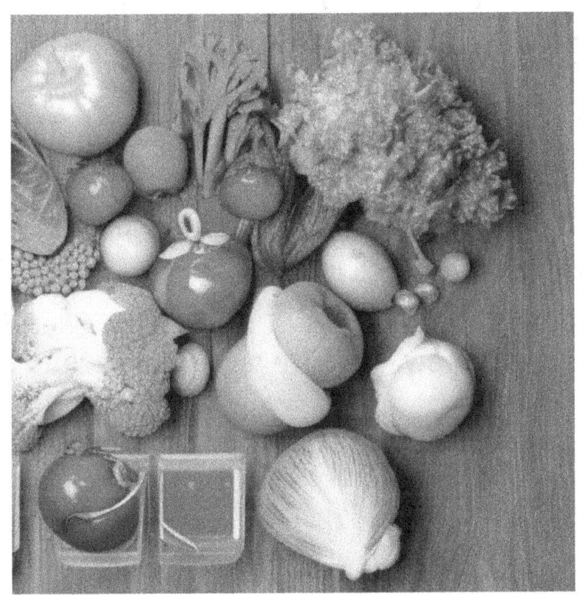

### Dr Ian Schmidt

Table Of Content

# Introduction

Lydia had always been an adventurous foodie, but her love for rich and spicy foods had taken a toll on her health. She had been experiencing frequent digestive issues and had been diagnosed with gallstones, a common condition that affects the gallbladder.

Her doctor advised her to make some dietary changes to improve her digestion and gallbladder health. Lydia was determined to take control of her health and started looking for ways to improve her diet.

One day, while browsing through a bookstore, she stumbled upon Dr Ian's gallbladder diet cookbook. The book contained a variety of delicious and healthy recipes that were specifically designed to support gallbladder health.

Excited by the prospect of a new and healthy culinary adventure, Lydia decided to give the cookbook a try. She started by preparing a few simple recipes, such as roasted chicken with steamed vegetables and quinoa salad with fresh herbs.

Lydia was pleasantly surprised at how easy and tasty the recipes were. She enjoyed experimenting with different spices and flavors and found that she didn't miss her old high-fat and spicy diet at all.

As she continued to cook from the cookbook, Lydia noticed a significant improvement in her digestive health. Her symptoms, including bloating and abdominal pain, began to subside, and she felt more energetic and focused.

With the help of the gallbladder diet cookbook, Lydia was able to take control of her health and enjoy a delicious and satisfying diet. She was grateful for the cookbook and the positive impact it had on her life.

**The gallbladder** is a small, pear-shaped organ located on the right side of the abdomen, just below the liver. Its main function is to store and concentrate bile, a greenish-yellow liquid produced by the liver that aids in the digestion of fats.

The gallbladder is connected to the liver and small intestine by a series of tubes that allow bile to flow from the liver to the gallbladder and from the gallbladder to the small intestine. When you eat a fatty meal, the gallbladder contracts and releases bile into the small intestine where it breaks down fat molecules into smaller particles for easier absorption by the body.

The gallbladder is a non-essential organ and you can live without it. However, when the gallbladder is removed, the liver still produces bile, but it is no longer stored and concentrated in the gallbladder. Afterward, it can cause digestive problems.

Gallstones are a common problem that can affect the gallbladder. They are small, hard deposits that accumulate in the gallbladder and can cause pain and inflammation. Gallstones can be treated with medication or surgery, depending on their size and severity. In summary, the gallbladder is a small but vital organ that plays an important role in fat digestion. You can live without a gallbladder, but it can cause digestive problems.

A healthy diet is essential to maintaining a healthy gallbladder. The gallbladder plays an important role in the digestion of fats, and certain foods can increase your risk of gallbladder problems such as gallstones and inflammation.

<u>Here are some dietary tips to help maintain a healthy gallbladder:</u>

1. *Eat a diet rich in fruits and vegetables*
Fruits and vegetables are rich in fiber and antioxidants, which help reduce inflammation in the body and prevent the formation of gallstones.

2. *Limit your intake of saturated and trans fats*
Foods high in saturated and trans fats, such as fried foods, processed meats, and high-fat dairy, may increase your risk of gallbladder

problems. Be selective and choose low-fat dairy products.

 3. *Avoid rapid weight loss or weight gain*
Rapid weight loss or weight gain can increase the risk of gallstone formation. If you need to lose weight, do it slowly and steadily over time, avoiding drastic or quick diets.

4. *Drink enough water*
Drinking plenty of water can help flush toxins out of your body and prevent gallstones from forming.

5. *Limit your intake of refined carbohydrates and sugar*
Refined carbohydrates and foods high in sugar, such as white bread, pasta, and sugary drinks, can increase your risk of inflammation and gallbladder problems.

6. *Incorporate healthy fats into your diet*
Foods high in healthy fats such as avocados, nuts and olive oil can help reduce inflammation and promote gallbladder health.

In summary, a healthy diet high in fruits and vegetables, low in saturated and trans fats, and high in water and healthy fats is essential to maintaining a healthy gallbladder. By making dietary changes, you can reduce your risk of gallbladder problems and maintain optimal digestive health.

Nourishing Recipes for a Healthy Gallbladder Cookbook is an excellent resource for people who want to maintain a healthy gallbladder through dietary changes. This cookbook is low in saturated and trans fats and contains fiber and antioxidants. We offer a variety of delicious, nutritious recipes designed to promote optimal digestive health.

**Here are some tips for using nutrition recipes from the Healthy Gallbladder Cookbook:**

*Meal plan:*
Plan your meals for the week before you start cooking. Flip through cookbooks, pick your favorite recipes, and make a shopping list of the ingredients you need.

*Read the recipe carefully:*
Before you start cooking, read the recipe carefully to make sure you have all the necessary ingredients and equipment, and understand the instructions. Follow the recipe: While it's tempting to modify or substitute recipes, it's important to follow the recipe exactly as written so that the dish is as successful as it was intended.

*Try new ingredients:*
Nutritional recipes for a healthy gallbladder cookbook include a variety of ingredients, some of which you've never used before. Add variety and nutrition to your diet.

*Please note the portion size:*
While the cookbook recipes are healthy and nutritious, it's important to be mindful of portion sizes to avoid overeating and maintain a healthy weight.

*Enjoy the process:*
Cooking is a fun activity. Take the time to prepare healthy and delicious meals for yourself

and your loved ones. In summary, the Nutrition Recipes for a Healthy Gallbladder Cookbook is a valuable resource for anyone trying to maintain a healthy gallbladder through dietary changes. Get the most out of this cookbook by following the tips above and enjoy good health.

# Breakfast Recipes

*Veggie Scramble:*
Ingredients:
1/2 onion, diced
1/2 red pepper, diced
1/4 cup mushrooms, diced
1/4 cup spinach, chopped
1/4 cup tomatoes, diced
1/4 cup cooked black beans
1/4 cup cooked quinoa
1 tsp. olive oil
sea salt and black pepper to taste

Instructions:
1. In a large skillet, heat olive oil over medium heat.
2. Add onion, red pepper, mushrooms, and spinach. Cook until vegetables are soft, about 5 minutes.
3. Add black beans, quinoa, tomatoes, and salt and pepper to taste. Cook for an additional 5 minutes.

4. Serve in a warm tortilla wrap, or enjoy as is.
Prep Time: 10 minutes
Cook Time: 10 minutes


*Blueberry Quinoa Parfait*
Ingredients:
1/2 cup cooked quinoa
1/2 cup blueberries
1/4 cup plain yogurt
1 tsp. honey

Instructions:
1. In a small bowl, combine cooked quinoa, blueberries, yogurt, and honey.
2. Serve in a parfait glass, or enjoy as is.
Prep Time: 5 minutes
Cook Time: 5 minutes


*Fruit and Nut Oatmeal*
Ingredients:
1/2 cup old-fashioned oats
1/2 cup almond milk
1/4 cup chopped walnuts
1/4 cup raisins
1/4 cup dried cranberries
1/4 tsp. ground cinnamon

Instructions:

1. In a small saucepan, combine oats, almond milk, walnuts, raisins, cranberries, and cinnamon.

2. Cook over medium heat, stirring occasionally, until oats are cooked through and liquid is absorbed.

3. Serve warm, or enjoy as is.

Prep Time: 5 minutes

Cook Time: 10 minutes

*Veggie Omelet*

Ingredients:

3 eggs

1/4 cup diced onion

1/4 cup diced red pepper

1/4 cup diced green pepper

1/4 cup diced mushrooms

1/4 cup chopped spinach

1/4 cup shredded cheese

sea salt and black pepper to taste

Instructions:

1. In a large bowl, whisk together eggs, onion, red pepper, green pepper, mushrooms, spinach, and cheese.
2. Season with salt and pepper to taste.
3. In a medium skillet, cook egg mixture over medium heat until omelet is cooked through and cheese is melted.
4. Serve immediately.
Prep Time: 10 minutes
Cook Time: 10 minutes

### *Toast with Avocado and Tomato*
Ingredients:
1 slice whole wheat toast
1/2 avocado, mashed
1/4 cup diced tomatoes
sea salt and black pepper to taste

Instructions:
1. Toast whole wheat toast.
2. Spread mashed avocado over toast.
3. Top with diced tomatoes and salt and pepper to taste.
4. Enjoy immediately.
Prep Time: 5 minutes
Cook Time: 5 minutes

## *Green Smoothie*

Ingredients:
1 cup spinach
1/2 banana
1/4 cup mango
1/4 cup pineapple
1/4 cup orange juice

Instructions:
1. In a blender, combine spinach, banana, mango, pineapple, and orange juice.
2. Blend until smooth.
3. Serve immediately.
Prep Time: 5 minutes
Cook Time: 5 minutes

## *Yogurt and Fruit Parfait*

Ingredients:
1/2 cup plain yogurt
1/2 cup chopped fruit (strawberries, blueberries, raspberries, etc.)
1/4 cup granola

Instructions:
1. In a parfait glass, layer yogurt, chopped fruit, and granola.

2. Serve immediately.
Prep Time: 5 minutes
Cook Time: 5 minutes

*Peanut Butter and Jelly Toast*
Ingredients:
1 slice whole wheat toast
1 tbsp. peanut butter
1 tbsp. jelly

Instructions:
1. Toast whole wheat toast.
2. Spread peanut butter over toast.
3. Spread jelly over peanut butter.
4. Enjoy immediately.
Prep Time: 5 minutes
Cook Time: 5 minutes

*Scrambled Eggs*
Ingredients:
2 eggs
1/4 cup diced onion
1/4 cup diced red pepper
1/4 cup diced green pepper
1/4 cup diced mushrooms
1/4 cup chopped spinach

sea salt and black pepper to taste

Instructions:
1. In a large skillet, whisk together eggs, onion, red pepper, green pepper, mushrooms, and spinach.
2. Season with salt and pepper to taste.
3. Cook over medium heat, stirring occasionally, until eggs are cooked through.
4. Serve immediately.
Prep Time: 10 minutes
Cook Time: 10 minutes

### *Oatmeal*
Ingredients:
1/2 cup old-fashioned oats
1 cup water
1/4 cup raisins
1/4 cup chopped walnuts
1/4 tsp. ground cinnamon

Instructions:
1. In a small saucepan, combine oats, water, raisins, walnuts, and cinnamon.

2. Cook over medium heat, stirring occasionally, until oats are cooked through and liquid is absorbed.

3. Serve warm, or enjoy as is.

Prep Time: 5 minutes

Cook Time: 10 minutes

## *Toast with Hummus and Tomato*

Ingredients:

1 slice whole wheat toast

1/4 cup hummus

1/4 cup diced tomatoes

sea salt and black pepper to taste

Instructions:

1. Toast whole wheat toast.

2. Spread hummus over toast.

3. Top with diced tomatoes and salt and pepper to taste.

4. Enjoy immediately.

Prep Time: 5 minutes

Cook Time: 5 minutes

## *Fruit and Nut Cereal*

Ingredients:

1/2 cup cereal

1/2 cup almond milk
1/4 cup chopped walnuts
1/4 cup raisins
1/4 cup dried cranberries
1/4 tsp. ground cinnamon

Instructions:
1. In a small bowl, combine cereal, almond milk, walnuts, raisins, cranberries, and cinnamon.
2. Serve in a cereal bowl, or enjoy as is.
Prep Time: 5 minutes
Cook Time: 5 minutes

### *Scrambled Tofu*
Ingredients:
1/2 block firm tofu, crumbled
1/4 cup diced onion
1/4 cup diced red pepper
1/4 cup diced green pepper
1/4 cup diced mushrooms
1/4 cup chopped spinach
sea salt and black pepper to taste

Instructions:

1. In a large skillet, scramble crumbled tofu with onion, red pepper, green pepper, mushrooms, and spinach.

2. Season with salt and pepper to taste.

3. Cook over medium heat, stirring occasionally, until tofu is cooked through.

4. Serve immediately.

Prep Time: 10 minutes

Cook Time: 10 minutes


### *Toast with Avocado and Egg*

Ingredients:

1 slice whole wheat toast

1/2 avocado, mashed

1 egg


Instructions:

1. Toast whole wheat toast.

2. Spread mashed avocado over toast.

3. Fry egg in a small skillet over medium heat until cooked through.

4. Place egg on top of avocado toast.

5. Enjoy immediately.

Prep Time: 5 minutes

Cook Time: 10 minutes

## _Oatmeal with Berries_

Ingredients:

1/2 cup rolled oats

1 cup water

1/2 cup mixed berries (fresh or frozen)

1 tablespoon honey

1 tablespoon chopped walnuts

Instructions:

-In a saucepan, bring the water to a boil.

-Add the oats and reduce the heat to low. Cook for 5 minutes, stirring occasionally.

-Add the berries and cook for an additional 2-3 minutes.

-Remove from heat and stir in the honey and walnuts.

-Serve immediately, while the oatmeal is still warm and the berries are juicy.

## _Greek Yogurt with Fruit and Nuts:_

Ingredients:

1 cup plain Greek yogurt

1/2 cup mixed fruit (fresh or frozen)

1 tablespoon honey

1 tablespoon chopped almonds

Instructions:
-In a bowl, mix together the yogurt and honey.
-Top with fruit and almonds.


*Scrambled Eggs with Spinach*
Ingredients:
2 eggs
1 cup fresh spinach
1/2 tablespoon olive oil
Salt and pepper to taste


Instructions:
-Rinse the spinach thoroughly and pat it dry with a paper towel. Then, roughly chop the spinach leaves into smaller pieces.
-Heat the olive oil in a skillet over medium-high heat.
-Once the skillet is hot, add the chopped spinach to the skillet and cook until it wilts down, stirring occasionally. This should take about 2-3 minutes.
-While the spinach is cooking, crack the eggs into a bowl and beat them until they are well mixed.
-Once the spinach has wilted down, pour the beaten eggs into the skillet with the spinach.

-Use a spatula to gently scramble the eggs, stirring occasionally, until they are cooked to your liking. This should take about 2-3 minutes. Season the scrambled eggs with salt and pepper to taste.

-Once the eggs are cooked, remove the skillet from the heat and serve the scrambled eggs with spinach hot. Enjoy!

## *Breakfast Smoothie*

Ingredients:

1/2 cup frozen mixed berries

1/2 banana

1/2 cup plain Greek yogurt

1/2 cup almond milk

1/2 tablespoon honey

Instructions:

-In a blender, combine all ingredients.

-Blend until smooth.

## *Cottage Cheese with Pineapple*

Ingredients:

1/2 cup cottage cheese

1/2 cup fresh pineapple

1 tablespoon chopped pecans

Instructions:
-In a bowl, mix together the cottage cheese and pineapple.
-Top with pecans.


*Sweet Potato Hash with Poached Eggs*
Ingredients:
1 sweet potato, peeled and diced
1/2 tablespoon olive oil
2 eggs
Salt and pepper to taste

Instructions:
-In a skillet, heat the olive oil over medium-high heat.
-Add the sweet potato and cook until tender. Season with salt and pepper.
-In a separate pot, bring water to a boil.
-Crack the eggs into the boiling water and cook until poached.
-Serve the sweet potato hash topped with poached eggs.


*Chia Seed Pudding*
Ingredients:
1/4 cup chia seeds

1 cup almond milk
1/2 tablespoon honey
1/4 teaspoon vanilla extract

Instructions:
-In a bowl, mix together the chia seeds, almond milk, honey, and vanilla extract.
-Refrigerate for at least 2 hours, or overnight.
-Serve chilled.

# Appetizers and Snacks

*Hummus & Veggie Platter*

Ingredients: 1 can chickpeas, 2 tablespoons olive oil, 2 tablespoons lemon juice, 1 tablespoon tahini, 1 garlic clove, 1 teaspoon cumin, 1 teaspoon smoked paprika, 1 pinch of salt, 1 cup of cucumbers, 1 cup of carrots.

Instructions: Drain and rinse the chickpeas. Place them in a blender with the olive oil, lemon juice, tahini, garlic, cumin, smoked paprika, and salt. Blend until smooth. Slice cucumbers and carrots into sticks and arrange on a platter. Serve with the hummus.
Preparation Method: Blending and slicing
Prep Time: 10 minutes

*Baked Sweet Potato Fries*

Ingredients: 2 large sweet potatoes, 2 tablespoons olive oil, 1 teaspoon smoked paprika, 1 teaspoon garlic powder, 1/2 teaspoon salt.

Instructions: Preheat oven to 400F. Peel and cut sweet potatoes into matchsticks. Place on a baking sheet. Drizzle with olive oil, smoked paprika, garlic powder, and salt. Bake for 25 minutes, flipping halfway through.
Preparation Method: Baking
Prep Time: 35 minutes

### Avocado Toast

Ingredients: 2 slices of whole wheat bread, 1 avocado, 1/4 teaspoon garlic powder, 1/4 teaspoon salt, 1 tablespoon extra-virgin olive oil, 2 tablespoons fresh chopped cilantro
Instructions: Toast the bread. Mash the avocado in a bowl with garlic powder, salt, olive oil, and cilantro. Spread the mashed avocado on the toast.
Preparation Method: Toasting, mashing
Prep Time: 10 minutes

### Greek Yogurt Dip

Ingredients: 1 cup plain Greek yogurt, 2 tablespoons olive oil, 1 tablespoon lemon juice, 1 teaspoon garlic powder, 1/2 teaspoon salt

Instructions: Mix all the ingredients together in a bowl. Serve with veggies or whole wheat crackers.

Preparation Method: Mixing

Prep Time: 5 minutes


## Baked Apple Chips

Ingredients: 2 apples, 1 teaspoon ground cinnamon, 1 tablespoon honey

Instructions: Preheat the oven to 350 degrees F. Slice the apples into thin slices. Place on a baking sheet. Sprinkle with cinnamon and honey. Bake for 15-20 minutes, flipping halfway through.

Preparation Method: Baking

Prep Time: 25 minutes


## Quinoa Veggie Bowl

Ingredients: 1 cup cooked quinoa, 1 cup chopped vegetables (such as peppers, onions, and mushrooms), 2 tablespoons olive oil, 1 teaspoon garlic powder, 1 teaspoon smoked paprika, 1/2 teaspoon salt

Instructions: Heat the olive oil in a large skillet. Add the vegetables and sauté until tender. Add the cooked quinoa, garlic powder, smoked

paprika, and salt. Cook until heated through. Serve in a bowl.
Preparation Method: Sautéing
Prep Time: 15 minutes


## Baked Zucchini Chips

Ingredients: 2 zucchini, 2 tablespoons olive oil, 1 teaspoon garlic powder, 1 teaspoon smoked paprika, 1/2 teaspoon salt
Instructions: Preheat the oven to 400 degrees F. Slice the zucchini into thin slices. Place on a baking sheet. Drizzle with olive oil, garlic powder, smoked paprika, and salt. Bake for 20 minutes, flipping halfway through.
Preparation Method: Baking
Prep Time: 25 minutes


## Roasted Chickpeas

Ingredients: 1 can chickpeas, 2 tablespoons olive oil, 1 teaspoon garlic powder, 1 teaspoon smoked paprika, 1/2 teaspoon salt
Instructions: Preheat the oven to 400 degrees F. Drain and rinse the chickpeas. Place on a baking sheet and drizzle with olive oil, garlic powder, smoked paprika, and salt. Bake for 25 minutes, flipping halfway through.

Preparation Method: Baking
Prep Time: 30 minutes

## *Cucumber & Tomato Salad*

Ingredients: 2 cucumbers, 1 tomato, 2 tablespoons olive oil, 1 tablespoon lemon juice, 1 teaspoon garlic powder, 1 teaspoon smoked paprika, 1/2 teaspoon salt

Instructions: Slice the cucumbers and tomato into thin slices. Place in a bowl and drizzle with olive oil, lemon juice, garlic powder, smoked paprika, and salt. Toss to combine.

Preparation Method: Slicing
Prep Time: 10 minutes

## *Baked Parmesan Sweet Potato Fries*

Ingredients: 2 large sweet potatoes, 2 tablespoons olive oil, 1/4 cup grated Parmesan cheese, 1 teaspoon garlic powder, 1 teaspoon smoked paprika, 1/2 teaspoon salt

Instructions: Preheat the oven to 400 degrees F. Peel and cut the sweet potatoes into matchsticks. Place on a baking sheet. Drizzle with olive oil, Parmesan cheese, garlic powder, smoked paprika, and salt. Bake for 25 minutes, flipping halfway through.

Preparation Method: Baking
Prep Time: 35 minutes


_Roasted Red Pepper Hummus_
Ingredients:
1 can chickpeas, drained and rinsed
1 roasted red pepper, chopped
2 tbsp tahini
2 cloves garlic, minced
2 tbsp lemon juice
2 tbsp olive oil
Salt and pepper to taste

Instructions:
-Add all ingredients to a food processor.
-Blend until smooth.
-Serve with veggies or crackers.
Prep time: 10 minutes

_Baked Sweet Potato Wedges_
Ingredients:
2 sweet potatoes, cut into wedges
1 tbsp olive oil
1 tsp paprika
1/2 tsp garlic powder
1/2 tsp salt

Instructions:

-Preheat the oven to 400°F (200°C).

-Toss the sweet potato wedges with olive oil, paprika, garlic powder, and salt.

-Place on a baking sheet lined with parchment paper.

-Bake for 25-30 minutes, or until tender and crispy.

Prep time: 10 minutes


## *Greek Yogurt and Cucumber Dip*

Ingredients:

1 cup Greek yogurt

1/2 cucumber, grated

2 cloves garlic, minced

2 tbsp chopped fresh dill

Salt and pepper to taste


Instructions:

-Grate the cucumber and squeeze out any excess water.

-Mix the Greek yogurt, grated cucumber, garlic, dill, salt, and pepper in a bowl.

-Chill for 15 minutes.

-Serve cold with veggies or crackers.

Prep time: 10 minutes

*Turkey and Cheese Roll-Ups*
Ingredients:
4 slices turkey breast
4 slices cheese
1/2 cup baby spinach leaves

Instructions:
-Lay the turkey slices on a cutting board.
-Place a slice of cheese and a few baby spinach leaves on each slice.
-Roll up tightly.
-Slice into bite-sized pieces.
Prep time: 5 minutes

*Tomato and Basil Salad*
Ingredients:
2 cups cherry tomatoes, halved
1/4 cup chopped fresh basil
1 tbsp balsamic vinegar
1 tbsp olive oil
Salt and pepper to taste

Instructions:
-Combine all ingredients in a bowl.
Mix well.

-Chill for 15 minutes.
Serve cold.
Prep time: 10 minutes

*Cottage Cheese and Fruit Bowl*
Ingredients:
1 cup cottage cheese
1 cup mixed fruit (berries, chopped apple, banana)

Instructions:
-Wash and chop the fruit.
-Layer the cottage cheese and fruit in a bowl.
-Serve chilled.
Prep time: 10 minutes

*Veggie Egg Muffins*
Ingredients:
6 eggs
1/4 cup milk
1/2 cup chopped veggies (bell peppers, mushrooms, spinach)
Salt and pepper to taste

Instructions:
-Preheat the oven to 350°F (175°C).

-Whisk the eggs and milk in a bowl.
-Stir in the chopped veggies, salt, and pepper.
-Pour the mixture into a greased muffin tin.
-Bake for 20-25 minutes, or until cooked through.
Prep time: 15 minutes

### *Grilled Chicken Skewers with Yogurt Dip*

Ingredients:
1 lb boneless, skinless chicken breasts, cut into cubes
1 tbsp olive oil
1 tsp paprika
1 tsp garlic powder
Salt and pepper to taste
1 cup Greek yogurt
1 tbsp chopped fresh dill

Instructions:
-Preheat the grill to medium-high heat.
-Toss the chicken cubes with olive oil, paprika, garlic powder, salt, and pepper.
-Thread the chicken onto skewers.
-Grill the skewers for 8-10 minutes, or until cooked through.
-Mix the Greek yogurt and dill in a small bowl.

-Serve the skewers with the yogurt dip.
Prep time: 20 minutes

*Grilled Eggplant Roll-Ups*
Ingredients:
1 eggplant, sliced lengthwise
1/2 cup ricotta cheese
1/4 cup chopped fresh basil
1/4 cup grated Parmesan cheese
Salt and pepper to taste

Instructions:
-Preheat the grill to medium heat.
-Season the eggplant slices with salt and pepper.
-Grill the eggplant slices for 2-3 minutes on each side.
-Mix the ricotta cheese, chopped basil, and grated Parmesan cheese in a bowl.
-Spoon the cheese mixture onto each eggplant slice.
-Roll up the eggplant slices.
Serve warm.
Prep time: 15 minutes

*Edamame Hummus*

Ingredients:
1 cup shelled edamame
1/4 cup tahini
1/4 cup water
2 tbsp lemon juice
1 garlic clove, minced
1/2 tsp cumin
Salt and pepper to taste

Instructions:
-Cook the edamame in boiling water for 3-4 minutes.
-Drain the edamame and rinse with cold water.
-Add the edamame, tahini, water, lemon juice, garlic, cumin, salt, and pepper to a food processor.
-Blend until smooth.
-Serve chilled with veggies or crackers.
Prep time: 10 minutes

*Cucumber and Tuna Salad*
Ingredients:
1 can tuna, drained
1 cucumber, chopped
1/4 cup chopped red onion
1/4 cup chopped fresh dill

2 tbsp olive oil
1 tbsp lemon juice
Salt and pepper to taste

Instructions:
-Combine all ingredients in a bowl.
-Mix well.
-Chill for 15 minutes.
-Serve cold.
Prep time: 10 minutes

*Baked Salmon Bites*
Ingredients:
1 lb salmon, cut into small cubes
2 tbsp olive oil
1 tsp paprika
1 tsp garlic powder
1/2 tsp salt

Instructions:
-Preheat the oven to 400°F (200°C).
-Toss the salmon cubes with olive oil, paprika, garlic powder, and salt.
-Place on a baking sheet lined with parchment paper.

-Bake for 10-12 minutes, or until cooked through.
-Serve warm.
Prep time: 15 minutes


## *Roasted Red Pepper and Feta Dip*
Ingredients:
1 jar roasted red peppers, drained
1/2 cup crumbled feta cheese
2 tbsp olive oil
1 garlic clove, minced
1 tsp dried oregano
Salt and pepper to taste

Instructions:
-Add the roasted red peppers, feta cheese, olive oil, garlic, oregano, salt, and pepper to a food processor.
-Blend until smooth.
-Serve chilled with veggies or crackers.
Prep time: 10 minutes


## *Tomato and Mozzarella Skewers*
Ingredients:
Cherry tomatoes
Fresh mozzarella balls

Fresh basil leaves
Balsamic vinegar

Instructions:
-Wash the cherry tomatoes and basil leaves.
Skewer the cherry tomatoes, mozzarella balls, and basil leaves.
-Drizzle with balsamic vinegar.
-Serve chilled.
Prep time:

# Soups And Salad

*Carrot Ginger Soup*
Ingredients:
1 pound carrots, peeled and chopped
1 small onion, chopped
2 cloves garlic, minced
1-inch piece ginger, peeled and grated
4 cups vegetable broth
1 tablespoon olive oil
Salt and pepper to taste

Instructions:
-Heat the olive oil in a large pot over medium heat.
-Add the onion and garlic and cook until softened, about 5 minutes.
-Add the ginger and cook for another minute.
-Add the carrots and broth and bring to a boil.
-Reduce heat and simmer until the carrots are tender, about 20-25 minutes.
-Puree the soup with an immersion blender or in batches in a regular blender.
-Season with salt and pepper to taste.
-Serve hot.

Prep time: 10 minutes, Cook time: 30 minutes

_Lentil Soup_
Ingredients:
1 cup dried lentils, rinsed and drained
1 onion, chopped
2 cloves garlic, minced
2 carrots, peeled and chopped
2 stalks celery, chopped
4 cups vegetable broth
1 tablespoon olive oil
1 teaspoon cumin
Salt and pepper to taste

Instructions:
-Heat the olive oil in a large pot over medium heat.
-Add the onion and garlic and cook until softened, about 5 minutes.
-Add the carrots and celery and cook for another 5 minutes.
-Add the lentils, broth, cumin, salt, and pepper and bring to a boil.
-Reduce heat and simmer until the lentils are tender, about 30 minutes.
-Serve hot.

Prep time: 10 minutes, Cook time: 35 minutes

*Butternut Squash Soup*
Ingredients:
1 butternut squash, peeled and chopped
1 onion, chopped
2 cloves garlic, minced
4 cups vegetable broth
1 tablespoon olive oil
1/4 teaspoon nutmeg
Salt and pepper to taste

Instructions:
-Heat the olive oil in a large pot over medium heat.
-Add the onion and garlic and cook until softened, about 5 minutes.
-Add the butternut squash, broth, nutmeg, salt, and pepper and bring to a boil.
-Reduce heat and simmer until the squash is tender, about 20-25 minutes.
-Puree the soup with an immersion blender or in batches in a regular blender.
-Season with salt and pepper to taste.
-Serve hot.
Prep time: 10 minutes, Cook time: 30 minutes

*Creamy Broccoli Soup*
Ingredients:
1 head broccoli, chopped
1 onion, chopped
2 cloves garlic, minced
4 cups vegetable broth
1 tablespoon olive oil
1/2 cup plain Greek yogurt
Salt and pepper to taste

Instructions:
-Heat the olive oil in a large pot over medium heat.
-Add the onion and garlic and cook until softened, about 5 minutes.
-Add the broccoli and broth and bring to a boil.
-Reduce heat and simmer until the broccoli is tender, about 20-25 minutes.
-Puree the soup with an immersion blender or in batches in a regular blender.
-Stir in the Greek yogurt.
-Season with salt and pepper to taste.
-Serve

_Cauliflower Soup with Parsley and Garlic_
(Prep time: 10 minutes, Serves 6):
Ingredients:
- 1 head cauliflower, cut into florets
- 2 tablespoons olive oil
- 2 cloves garlic, minced
- 2 tablespoons fresh parsley, chopped
- 4 cups vegetable stock
- Salt and pepper, to taste

Instructions:
1. Heat a large pot over medium heat, add the olive oil and garlic and sauté for 1-2 minutes.
2. Add the cauliflower and sauté for another 2 minutes.
3. Add the vegetable stock and bring to a boil.
4. Reduce the heat to low and simmer for 10 minutes.
5. Add the parsley and season with salt and pepper.
6. Using an immersion blender, blend the soup until smooth.
7. Serve hot.

_Kale and Quinoa Salad_
(Prep time: 10 minutes, Serves 4):

Ingredients:
- 2 cups kale, chopped
- 1 cup cooked quinoa
- 1/2 cup cherry tomatoes, halved
- 1/4 cup feta cheese, crumbled
- 2 tablespoons olive oil
- 1 tablespoon lemon juice
- Salt and pepper, to taste

Instructions:
1. In a large bowl, combine the kale, quinoa, tomatoes and feta cheese.
2. In a small bowl, whisk together the olive oil and lemon juice.
3. Pour the dressing over the salad and toss to combine.
4. Season with salt and pepper, to taste.
5. Serve chilled.

*White Bean and Spinach Soup*
(Prep time: 15 minutes, Serves 4):
Ingredients:
- 2 tablespoons olive oil
- 1 onion, diced
- 2 cloves garlic, minced
- 2 cups vegetable stock

- 1 15-ounce can white beans, drained and rinsed
- 4 cups baby spinach
- Salt and pepper, to taste

Instructions:
1. Heat a large pot over medium heat, add the olive oil and onion and sauté for 3 minutes.
2. Add the garlic and sauté for another minute.
3. Add the vegetable stock and bring to a boil.
4. Reduce the heat to low and add the white beans. Simmer for 10 minutes.
5. Add the spinach and cook for another 2 minutes.
6. Using an immersion blender, blend the soup until smooth.
7. Season with salt and pepper, to taste.
8. Serve hot.

_Avocado and Tomato Salad_
(Prep time: 5 minutes, Serves 4):
Ingredients:
- 1 avocado, diced
- 2 tomatoes, diced
- 1/2 red onion, diced
- 2 tablespoons olive oil

- 1 tablespoon lemon juice
- Salt and pepper, to taste

Instructions:
1. In a large bowl, combine the avocado, tomatoes, and red onion.
2. In a small bowl, whisk together the olive oil and lemon juice.
3. Pour the dressing over the salad and toss to combine.
4. Season with salt and pepper, to taste.
5. Serve chilled.

## *Roasted Carrot Soup*
(Prep time: 20 minutes, Serves 4):
Ingredients:
- 1 pound carrots, peeled and chopped
- 2 tablespoons olive oil
- 1 onion, diced
- 2 cloves garlic, minced
- 4 cups vegetable broth
- Salt and pepper, to taste

Instructions:
1. Preheat oven to 400°F.

2. Place the carrots on a baking sheet and drizzle with olive oil.

3. Roast in the oven for 20 minutes, or until the carrots are tender.

4. Heat a large pot over medium heat, add the olive oil and onion and sauté for 3 minutes.

5. Add the garlic and sauté for another minute.

6. Add the roasted carrots and vegetable broth and bring to a boil.

7. Reduce the heat to low and simmer for 10 minutes.

8. Using an immersion blender, blend the soup until smooth.

9. Season with salt and pepper, to taste.

10. Serve hot.

### _Roasted Butternut Squash Salad_
(Prep time: 20 minutes, Serves 4):
Ingredients:
- 1 butternut squash, peeled and cubed
- 2 tablespoons olive oil
- 1/2 cup walnuts, chopped
- 1/4 cup dried cranberries
- 2 tablespoons balsamic vinegar
- Salt and pepper, to taste

Instructions:

1. Preheat oven to 400°F.

2. Place the butternut squash on a baking sheet and drizzle with olive oil.

3. Roast in the oven for 20 minutes, or until the squash is tender.

4. In a large bowl, combine the roasted squash, walnuts and cranberries.

5. Drizzle with the balsamic vinegar and toss to combine.

6. Season with salt and pepper, to taste.

7. Serve chilled.


*Lentil Soup with Kale and Sweet Potatoes*

(Prep time: 20 minutes, Serves 4):

Ingredients:

- 2 tablespoons olive oil
- 1 onion, diced
- 2 cloves garlic, minced
- 2 cups vegetable broth
- 1 cup lentils, rinsed
- 1 sweet potato, peeled and cubed
- 2 cups kale, chopped
- Salt and pepper, to taste


Instructions:

1. Heat a large pot over medium heat, add the olive oil and onion and sauté for 3 minutes.
2. Add the garlic and sauté for another minute.
3. Add the vegetable broth, lentils, and sweet potato and bring to a boil.
4. Reduce the heat to low and simmer for 10 minutes.
5. Add the kale and simmer for another 5 minutes.
6. Using an immersion blender, blend the soup until smooth.
7. Season with salt and pepper, to taste.
8. Serve hot.

*Fennel and Apple Salad*
 (Prep time: 10 minutes, Serves 4):
Ingredients:
- 2 fennel bulbs, thinly sliced
- 2 apples, cored and thinly sliced
- 2 tablespoons olive oil
- 1 tablespoon lemon juice
- 2 tablespoons fresh parsley, chopped
- Salt and pepper, to taste

Instructions:

1. In a large bowl, combine the fennel and apples.

2. In a small bowl, whisk together the olive oil and lemon juice.

3. Pour the dressing over the salad and toss to combine.

4. Add the parsley and season with salt and pepper, to taste.

5. Serve chilled.


*Mushroom and Spinach Soup*
(Prep time: 10 minutes, Serves 4):
Ingredients:
- 2 tablespoons olive oil
- 1 onion, diced
- 2 cloves garlic, minced
- 1 pound mushrooms, sliced
- 4 cups vegetable broth
- 4 cups baby spinach
- Salt and pepper, to taste

Instructions:
1. Heat a large pot over medium heat, add the olive oil and onion and sauté for 3 minutes.

2. Add the garlic and mushrooms and sauté for another 2 minutes.

3. Add the vegetable broth and bring to a boil.

4. Reduce the heat to low and simmer for 10 minutes.

5. Add the spinach and cook for another 2 minutes.

6. Using an immersion blender, blend the soup until smooth.

7. Season with salt and pepper, to taste.

8. Serve hot.

## *Beet and Carrot Salad*

(Prep time: 10 minutes, Serves 4):

Ingredients:

- 2 beets, peeled and grated
- 2 carrots, grated
- 2 tablespoons olive oil
- 1 tablespoon lemon juice
- 2 tablespoons fresh parsley, chopped
- Salt and pepper, to taste

Instructions:

1. In a large bowl, combine the beets and carrots.

2. In a small bowl, whisk together the olive oil and lemon juice.

3. Pour the dressing over the salad and toss to combine.

4. Add the parsley and season with salt and pepper, to taste.

5. Serve chilled.

## *Cucumber and Tomato Salad*

(Prep time: 5 minutes, Serves 4):

Ingredients:

- 2 cucumbers, diced
- 2 tomatoes, diced
- 2 tablespoons olive oil
- 1 tablespoon lemon juice
- 2 tablespoons fresh parsley, chopped
- Salt and pepper, to taste

Instructions:

1. In a large bowl, combine the cucumbers and tomatoes.

2. In a small bowl, whisk together the olive oil and lemon juice.

3. Pour the dressing over the salad and toss to combine.

4. Add the parsley and season with salt and pepper, to taste.

5. Serve chilled.

*<u>White Bean and Spinach Soup</u>*
(Prep time: 15 minutes, Serves 4):
Ingredients:
- 2 tablespoons olive oil
- 1 onion, diced
- 2 cloves garlic, minced
- 2 cups vegetable stock
- 1 15-ounce can white beans, drained and rinsed
- 4 cups baby spinach
- Salt and pepper, to taste

Instructions:
1. Heat a large pot over medium heat, add the olive oil and onion and sauté for 3 minutes.
2. Add the garlic and sauté for another minute.
3. Add the vegetable stock and bring to a boil.
4. Reduce the heat to low and add the white beans. Simmer for 10 minutes.
5. Add the spinach and cook for another 2 minutes.
6. Using an immersion blender, blend the soup until smooth.
7. Season with salt and pepper, to taste.

8. Serve hot.

*Lentil Soup with Kale and Sweet Potatoes*
(Prep time: 20 minutes, Serves 4):
Ingredients:
- 2 tablespoons olive oil
- 1 onion, diced
- 2 cloves garlic, minced
- 2 cups vegetable broth
- 1 cup lentils, rinsed
- 1 sweet potato, peeled and cubed
- 2 cups kale, chopped
- Salt and pepper, to taste

Instructions:
1. Heat a large pot over medium heat, add the olive oil and onion and sauté for 3 minutes.
2. Add the garlic and sauté for another minute.
3. Add the vegetable broth, lentils, and sweet potato and bring to a boil.
4. Reduce the heat to low and simmer for 10 minutes.
5. Add the kale and simmer for another 5 minutes.
6. Using an immersion blender, blend the soup until smooth.

7. Season with salt and pepper, to taste.
8. Serve hot.


*Fennel and Apple Salad*
 (Prep time: 10 minutes, Serves 4):
Ingredients:
- 2 fennel bulbs, thinly sliced
- 2 apples, cored and thinly sliced
- 2 tablespoons olive oil
- 1 tablespoon lemon juice
- 2 tablespoons fresh parsley, chopped
- Salt and pepper, to taste

Instructions:
1. In a large bowl, combine the fennel and apples.
2. In a small bowl, whisk together the olive oil and lemon juice.
3. Pour the dressing over the salad and toss to combine.
4. Add the parsley and season with salt and pepper, to taste.
5. Serve chilled.


*Mushroom and Spinach Soup*
 (Prep time: 10 minutes, Serves 4):

Ingredients:
- 2 tablespoons olive oil
- 1 onion, diced
- 2 cloves garlic, minced
- 1 pound mushrooms, sliced
- 4 cups vegetable broth
- 4 cups baby spinach
- Salt and pepper, to taste

Instructions:
1. Heat a large pot over medium heat, add the olive oil and onion and sauté for 3 minutes.
2. Add the garlic and mushrooms and sauté for another 2 minutes.
3. Add the vegetable broth and bring to a boil.
4. Reduce the heat to low and simmer for 10 minutes.
5. Add the spinach and cook for another 2 minutes.
6. Using an immersion blender, blend the soup until smooth.
7. Season with salt and pepper, to taste.
8. Serve hot.

### *Beet and Carrot Salad*
(Prep time: 10 minutes, Serves 4):

Ingredients:
- 2 beets, peeled and grated
- 2 carrots, grated
- 2 tablespoons olive oil
- 1 tablespoon lemon juice
- 2 tablespoons fresh parsley, chopped
- Salt and pepper, to taste

Instructions:
1. In a large bowl, combine the beets and carrots.
2. In a small bowl, whisk together the olive oil and lemon juice.
3. Pour the dressing over the salad and toss to combine.
4. Add the parsley and season with salt and pepper, to taste.
5. Serve chilled.

### *Split Pea Soup with Bacon*
(Prep time: 20 minutes, Serves 4):
Ingredients:
- 4 slices bacon, diced
- 1 onion, diced
- 2 cloves garlic, minced
- 1 pound split peas, rinsed

- 4 cups vegetable broth
- Salt and pepper, to taste

Instructions:
1. Heat a large pot over medium heat, add the bacon and sauté for 5 minutes.
2. Add the onion and garlic and sauté for another 3 minutes.
3. Add the split peas and vegetable broth and bring to a boil.
4. Reduce the heat to low and simmer for 15 minutes.
5. Using an immersion blender, blend the soup until smooth.
6. Season with salt and pepper, to taste.
7. Serve hot.

*Mediterranean Salad*
Ingredients:
4 cups mixed greens
1 cucumber, chopped
1 tomato, chopped
1/4 cup chopped red onion
1/4 cup crumbled feta cheese
1/4 cup kalamata olives
2 tbsp extra-virgin olive oil

1 tbsp red wine vinegar
Salt and pepper to taste

Instructions:
-In a large bowl, combine the mixed greens, cucumber, tomato, red onion, feta cheese, and olives.
-Drizzle with olive oil and red wine vinegar.
-Season with salt and pepper to taste.
-Toss to combine and serve.
Prep time: 10 minutes

*Grilled Chicken Salad*
Ingredients:
4 cups mixed greens
1 grilled chicken breast, sliced
1/2 cup cherry tomatoes, halved
1/2 cup chopped cucumber
1/4 cup chopped red onion
1/4 cup crumbled feta cheese
2 tbsp extra-virgin olive oil
1 tbsp balsamic vinegar
Salt and pepper to taste

Instructions:

-In a large bowl, combine the mixed greens, grilled chicken, cherry tomatoes, cucumber, red onion, and feta cheese.
-Drizzle with olive oil and balsamic vinegar.
-Season with salt and pepper to taste.
-Toss to combine and serve.
Prep time: 20 minutes


*Roasted Sweet Potato and Balsamic Beet Salad*
(prep time: 15 minutes)

Ingredients:
-3 large sweet potatoes, peeled and cubed
-3 beets, peeled and sliced
-2 tablespoons olive oil
-2 tablespoons balsamic vinegar
-Salt and pepper to taste
-1/2 cup feta cheese, crumbled
-1/4 cup toasted walnuts

Instructions:
1. Preheat oven to 400°F.
2. Place sweet potatoes and beets on a large baking sheet and drizzle with olive oil and

balsamic vinegar. Sprinkle with salt and pepper.

3. Roast for 15 minutes, stirring occasionally.

4. Remove from oven and let cool.

5. In a large bowl, combine roasted sweet potatoes and beets with feta cheese and toasted walnuts.

6. Serve immediately. Enjoy!


*Kale and Chickpea Salad*
(prep time: 10minutes)

Ingredients:
-4 cups kale, chopped
-1 can chickpeas, rinsed and drained
-1/2 cup red bell pepper, diced
-1/4 cup red onion, diced
-2 tablespoons olive oil
-1 tablespoon apple cider vinegar
-1/4 teaspoon garlic powder
-Salt and pepper to taste

Instructions:

1. In a large bowl, combine kale, chickpeas, bell pepper, and red onion.
2. In a small bowl, whisk together olive oil, apple cider vinegar, garlic powder, salt, and pepper.
3. Drizzle dressing over salad and toss to combine.
4. Serve immediately. Enjoy!

# Main Entrees

*Grilled Salmon with Roasted Vegetables*
Ingredients:
4 salmon fillets
2 cups mixed vegetables (bell peppers, zucchini, onion, carrots)
2 tbsp olive oil
Salt and pepper to taste

Instructions:
-Preheat grill to medium-high heat.
-Toss vegetables with olive oil, salt, and pepper.
-Place salmon and vegetables on grill.
-Cook salmon for 4-6 minutes per side or until it flakes easily with a fork.
-Cook vegetables for 10-12 minutes or until they are tender and slightly charred.
-Serve salmon and vegetables hot.
Prep time: 25 minutes

*Turkey and Vegetable Stir-Fry*

Ingredients:
1 pound ground turkey
2 cups mixed vegetables (broccoli, bell peppers, carrots, snap peas)
2 tbsp low-sodium soy sauce
1 tbsp honey
1 tbsp sesame oil
1 tbsp cornstarch
1 tbsp ginger, grated
Salt and pepper to taste

Instructions:
-Heat sesame oil in a large skillet over medium-high heat.
-Add ground turkey and cook until browned, about 5-7 minutes.
-Add vegetables and ginger, and cook for 5-7 minutes or until the vegetables are tender.
-In a small bowl, whisk together soy sauce, honey, and cornstarch.
-Pour the sauce over the turkey and vegetables, stirring until everything is coated.
-Cook for an additional 2-3 minutes, until the sauce thickens.
-Serve hot.
Prep time: 30 minutes

## *Broiled Chicken with Grilled Asparagus*

Ingredients:

4 boneless, skinless chicken breasts

1 lb asparagus, trimmed

2 tbsp olive oil

2 cloves garlic, minced

Salt and pepper to taste

Instructions:

-Preheat broiler.

-Place chicken on a baking sheet and season with salt and pepper.

-Broil chicken for 6-8 minutes per side or until it is cooked through.

-In a separate bowl, toss asparagus with olive oil, garlic, salt, and pepper.

-Grill asparagus on a preheated grill for 5-7 minutes or until tender and slightly charred.

-Serve chicken and asparagus hot.

Prep time: 25 minutes

## *Baked Tilapia with Quinoa Pilaf*

Ingredients:

4 tilapia fillets

1 cup quinoa, rinsed

2 cups chicken or vegetable broth
1 onion, chopped
2 cloves garlic, minced
1 tbsp olive oil
1 tsp paprika
Salt and pepper to taste

Instructions:
-Preheat oven to 375°F.
-In a large saucepan, heat olive oil over medium-high heat.
-Add onion and garlic, and sauté for 2-3 minutes or until the onion is translucent.
-Add quinoa, broth, paprika, salt, and pepper, and bring to a boil.
-Reduce heat to low, cover, and simmer for 15-20 minutes or until quinoa is cooked and liquid is absorbed.
-Place tilapia fillets on a baking sheet, and season with salt and pepper.
-Bake tilapia for 10-12 minutes or until it is cooked through.
-Serve tilapia with quinoa pilaf.
Prep time: 35 minutes

*Baked Chicken Breast with Mixed Vegetables*

Ingredients:
4 boneless, skinless chicken breasts
1 tbsp. olive oil
1/2 tsp. garlic powder
1/2 tsp. dried oregano
Salt and pepper
1 lb. mixed vegetables (broccoli, cauliflower, carrots, etc.)

Instructions:
-Preheat oven to 375°F.
-In a small bowl, mix together olive oil, garlic powder, oregano, salt, and pepper.
-Place chicken breasts in a baking dish and brush with the oil mixture.
-Bake chicken for 25-30 minutes, until cooked through.
-While chicken is cooking, toss mixed vegetables with a little bit of olive oil, salt, and pepper.
-Roast vegetables in the oven for 15-20 minutes, until tender.
-Serve chicken with vegetables on the side.
Prep time: 40 minutes

## Turkey Chili with Brown Rice

Ingredients:
1 lb. ground turkey
1 onion, chopped
1 green bell pepper, chopped
1 can (14 oz.) diced tomatoes
1 can (14 oz.) kidney beans, drained and rinsed
1 tbsp. chili powder
1 tsp. cumin
1/2 tsp. paprika
1/2 tsp. garlic powder
Salt and pepper
2 cups cooked brown rice

Instructions:
-In a large pot, brown ground turkey over medium-high heat.
-Add chopped onion and bell pepper and sauté until softened, about 5 minutes.
-Add diced tomatoes, kidney beans, chili powder, cumin, paprika, garlic powder, salt, and pepper. Stir to combine.
-Reduce heat to low and simmer for 20-25 minutes, until flavors have melded together.
-Serve chili over cooked brown rice.
Prep time: 40 minutes

<u>*Grilled Salmon with Roasted Brussels Sprouts*</u>
Ingredients:
4 salmon fillets
1 lemon, juiced
2 tbsp. olive oil
1 tsp. dried thyme
Salt and pepper
1 lb. Brussels sprouts, trimmed and halved
1 tbsp. olive oil
Salt and pepper

Instructions:
-Preheat grill to medium-high heat.
-In a small bowl, whisk together lemon juice, olive oil, thyme, salt, and pepper.
-Brush salmon fillets with the marinade and let sit for 15 minutes.
-Grill salmon for 6-8 minutes per side, until cooked through.
-Preheat oven to 375°F.
-Toss Brussels sprouts with olive oil, salt, and pepper.
-Roast Brussels sprouts in the oven for 20-25 minutes, until tender and slightly caramelized.
-Serve salmon with Brussels sprouts on the side.

Prep time: 40 minutes

*Grilled Salmon with Zucchini Noodles*
Ingredients:
4 salmon fillets
1 tbsp. olive oil
Salt and pepper
2 zucchinis, spiralized
1 tbsp. butter
1 clove garlic, minced
1/4 cup grated Parmesan cheese
Fresh parsley, chopped

Instructions:
-Preheat grill to medium-high heat.
-Brush salmon with olive oil and season with salt and pepper.
-Grill salmon for 5-6 minutes per side, until cooked through.
-In a large skillet, melt butter over medium heat.
-Add garlic and cook for 1 minute.
-Add zucchini noodles and cook for 2-3 minutes, until tender.
-Stir in Parmesan cheese and parsley.
Serve salmon on top of zucchini noodles.

Prep time: 20 minutes

*Baked Cod with Roasted Tomatoes and Green Beans*
Ingredients:
4 cod fillets
1 tbsp. olive oil
Salt and pepper
1 pint cherry tomatoes
1 lb. green beans
1 tbsp. olive oil
Salt and pepper

Instructions:
-Preheat the oven to 375°F.
-Place cod fillets in a baking dish and brush with olive oil. Season with salt and pepper.
-Scatter cherry tomatoes around the cod fillets.
-Bake for 15-20 minutes, until cod is cooked through.
-Trim ends of green beans and toss with olive oil, salt, and pepper.
-Roast green beans in the oven for 10-15 minutes, until tender.
-Serve cod with roasted tomatoes and green beans on the side.

Prep time: 25 minutes

*Turkey Chili with Sweet Potato*
Ingredients:
1 lb. ground turkey
1 tbsp. olive oil
1 onion, chopped
1 red bell pepper, chopped
1 tbsp. chili powder
1 tsp. cumin
1/2 tsp. paprika
1/4 tsp. cayenne pepper
1 can diced tomatoes
1 can black beans, drained and rinsed
1 large sweet potato, peeled and diced
Salt and pepper
Chopped cilantro (optional)

Instructions:
-In a large pot, heat olive oil over medium-high heat.
-Add ground turkey and cook until browned.
-Add onion and red bell pepper and cook until softened.
-Stir in chili powder, cumin, paprika, and cayenne pepper.

-Add diced tomatoes (including juice), black beans, and sweet potato. Season with salt and pepper.
-Bring to a boil, then reduce heat and simmer for 20-25 minutes, until sweet potato is tender.
-Serve chili topped with chopped cilantro, if desired.
Prep time: 30 minutes

*Lemon Garlic Shrimp and Zucchini Noodles*
Ingredients:
1 lb. shrimp, peeled and deveined
2 tbsp. olive oil
3 cloves garlic, minced
Juice of 1 lemon
1/4 tsp. red pepper flakes
Salt and pepper
4 medium zucchini, spiralized into noodles
Fresh parsley, chopped

Instructions:
-Heat olive oil in a large pan over medium-high heat.
-Add garlic and cook until fragrant.
-Add shrimp and cook until pink and cooked through.

-Add lemon juice, red pepper flakes, salt, and pepper. Stir to combine.
-Add zucchini noodles and cook until tender, about 3-5 minutes.
-Serve hot, garnished with fresh parsley.
Prep time: 20 minutes


_Baked Chicken and Vegetable Casserole_
Ingredients:
4 boneless, skinless chicken breasts
1 lb green beans, trimmed
2 cups baby carrots
2 cups diced red potatoes
1/4 cup olive oil
2 cloves garlic, minced
1 tsp dried thyme
Salt and pepper to taste

Instructions:
-Preheat the oven to 400°F.
-In a large bowl, toss together the green beans, baby carrots, and diced red potatoes with the olive oil, minced garlic, dried thyme, salt, and pepper.
-Spread the vegetable mixture in an even layer in a 9x13 inch baking dish.

-Arrange the chicken breasts on top of the vegetables.
-Season the chicken breasts with salt and pepper to taste.
-Bake the chicken and vegetable casserole in the preheated oven for 25-30 minutes, or until the chicken is cooked through and the vegetables are tender.
Prep time: 15 minutes
Cook time: 25-30 minutes

*Turkey Stuffed Peppers*
Ingredients:
4 bell peppers, halved and seeded
1 lb ground turkey
1 tbsp olive oil
1 onion, diced
2 cloves garlic, minced
1 zucchini, diced
1 cup cooked brown rice
1 cup low-sodium tomato sauce
1 tsp dried oregano
Salt and pepper to taste
1/2 cup shredded cheddar cheese

Instructions:

-Preheat oven to 375°F.

-Place the bell pepper halves in a baking dish and set aside.

-In a large skillet, heat olive oil over medium-high heat.

-Add onion and garlic, and cook until softened, about 5 minutes.

-Add ground turkey and cook until browned, breaking it up with a spoon.

-Add diced zucchini, cooked brown rice, tomato sauce, oregano, salt, and pepper. Stir to combine.

-Spoon the turkey mixture into the bell pepper halves.

-Cover with foil and bake for 30 minutes.

-Remove foil, sprinkle shredded cheddar cheese on top, and bake for an additional 10-15 minutes until cheese is melted and bubbly.

Prep time: 20 minutes

Cook time: 45 minutes

Total time: 65 minutes


*Broiled Salmon with Herb Butter*

Ingredients:

4 salmon fillets

2 tbsp unsalted butter, softened
2 tbsp chopped fresh parsley
1 tbsp chopped fresh chives
1 tbsp chopped fresh tarragon
1 tsp lemon zest
1/2 tsp salt
1/4 tsp black pepper

Instructions:
-Preheat the broiler to high.
-In a small bowl, mix together the butter, parsley, chives, tarragon, lemon zest, salt, and pepper.
-Place the salmon fillets on a baking sheet lined with parchment paper.
-Spread the herb butter over the salmon fillets.
-Broil the salmon for 7-10 minutes, or until the salmon is cooked through and the butter is melted and slightly browned.


### *Salmon with Asparagus and Lemon*
 Prep Time: 15 minutes
Ingredients:
• 4 (4-ounce) salmon fillets
• 1/2 teaspoon salt

- 1/4 teaspoon freshly ground black pepper
- 2 tablespoons olive oil
- 2 cloves garlic, minced
- 2 tablespoons freshly squeezed lemon juice
- 1/2 teaspoon dried oregano
- 1/4 teaspoon dried thyme
- 1/4 teaspoon red pepper flakes
- 2 bunches of fresh asparagus, trimmed

Instructions:
1. Preheat oven to 400°F.
2. Season salmon with salt and pepper.
3. Heat oil in an oven-safe skillet over medium heat.
4. Add garlic and cook until fragrant, about 1 minute.
5. Add salmon to the skillet and cook until lightly browned, 2 to 3 minutes.
6. Flip salmon and cook until almost cooked through, 2 to 3 minutes.
7. Add lemon juice, oregano, thyme, and red pepper flakes to the skillet.
8. Place asparagus around the salmon.
9. Transfer skillet to the oven and bake until salmon is cooked through and asparagus is tender, 8 to 10 minutes.

10. Serve salmon with asparagus and lemon sauce. Enjoy!

*Baked Falafel*
Ingredients:
2 cups cooked chickpeas
1 small onion, chopped
2 cloves garlic, minced
1/4 cup chopped fresh parsley
1/4 cup chopped fresh cilantro
2 tbsp whole wheat flour
1 tsp ground cumin
1 tsp ground coriander
Salt and pepper to taste
2 tbsp olive oil

Instructions:
-Preheat the oven to 375°F.
-In a food processor, pulse the chickpeas, onion, garlic, parsley, cilantro, flour, cumin, coriander, salt, and pepper until well combined.
-Form the mixture into small balls or patties.
-Brush a baking sheet with olive oil and place the falafel on the baking sheet.

-Bake for 20-25 minutes or until the falafel is golden brown and crispy.

*Chicken Shawarma*
Ingredients:
1 lb boneless, skinless chicken breast, sliced into thin strips
2 tbsp olive oil
2 cloves garlic, minced
1 tsp ground cumin
1 tsp paprika
1/2 tsp ground coriander
Salt and pepper to taste
4 pita breads
1 cup chopped lettuce
1 cup diced tomato
1/2 cup diced cucumber
1/4 cup chopped fresh parsley
1/4 cup chopped fresh mint
Tahini sauce for serving

Instructions:
-In a large bowl, combine the chicken strips, olive oil, garlic, cumin, paprika, coriander, salt, and pepper.

-Marinate the chicken in the refrigerator for at least 30 minutes.
-Preheat a grill or grill pan over medium-high heat.
-Grill the chicken strips for 3-4 minutes per side or until cooked through.
-Warm the pita breads on the grill.
-Stuff the pita breads with the grilled chicken, chopped lettuce, diced tomato, diced cucumber, parsley, mint, and tahini sauce.
-Serve immediately.

### *Mujadara (Lentils and Rice)*
Ingredients:
1 cup brown or green lentils, rinsed and drained
1 cup long-grain brown rice
2 tbsp olive oil
1 large onion, thinly sliced
1 tsp ground cumin
1 tsp ground coriander
Salt and pepper to taste

Instructions:
-In a large pot, bring 3 cups of water to a boil.
-Add the lentils and rice to the pot and stir.

-Reduce the heat to low and cover the pot.
-Simmer for 35-40 minutes or until the lentils and rice are cooked and the water has been absorbed.
-In a separate skillet, heat the olive oil over medium-high heat.
-Add the sliced onion to the skillet and sauté until caramelized and crispy.
-Add the cumin and coriander to the skillet and cook for another minute.
-Serve the mujadara topped with the caramelized onions.

*Beef and Vegetable Stir-Fry*
Ingredients:
1 lb beef strips
Salt and pepper to taste
2 tbsp olive oil
2 cloves garlic, minced
1 onion, chopped
1 red bell pepper, sliced
1 green bell pepper, sliced
1 cup broccoli florets
1 cup sliced mushrooms
1/4 cup low-sodium soy sauce

Instructions:

-Season the beef strips with salt and pepper.

-Heat the olive oil in a large wok or skillet over high heat.

-Add the minced garlic and chopped onion to the wok and cook until tender, stirring occasionally.

-Add the beef strips to the wok and cook until browned on all sides.

-Add the sliced bell peppers, broccoli florets, and sliced mushrooms to the wok and stir-fry for 3-5 minutes or until the vegetables are tender-crisp.

-Add the low-sodium soy sauce to the wok and stir to combine.

-Serve hot over brown rice or quinoa.

### *Lentil and Vegetable Bobotie*

Ingredients:

1 tbsp olive oil

1 onion, chopped

2 cloves garlic, minced

1 red bell pepper, chopped

2 carrots, peeled and chopped

1 zucchini, chopped

1 tsp ground cumin

1 tsp ground coriander
1 tsp turmeric
1/2 tsp cinnamon
Salt and pepper to taste
1 cup brown lentils, cooked
1/4 cup apricot jam
1/4 cup low-fat milk
2 eggs, beaten
1/4 cup almonds, chopped

Instructions:
-Preheat the oven to 350°F (180°C).
-In a large skillet, heat the olive oil over medium heat.
-Add the chopped onion and minced garlic to the skillet and cook until tender, stirring occasionally.
-Add the chopped red bell pepper, carrots, and zucchini to the skillet and cook until tender, stirring occasionally.
-Add the ground cumin, ground coriander, turmeric, cinnamon, salt, and pepper to the skillet and stir to combine.
-Stir in the cooked brown lentils, apricot jam, and low-fat milk to the skillet.

-Transfer the lentil and vegetable mixture to a 9-inch square baking dish.
-In a small bowl, beat the eggs and pour over the lentil and vegetable mixture.
-Sprinkle the chopped almonds over the top of the dish.
-Bake the dish for 30-35 minutes or until the top is golden brown and the eggs are set.
Serve hot.

# Sides And Beverages

*Roasted Brussels Sprouts*
Ingredients:
1 pound Brussels sprouts, trimmed and halved
1 tbsp olive oil
Salt and pepper to taste

Instructions:
-Preheat the oven to 400°F (200°C).
-Place the trimmed and halved Brussels sprouts on a baking sheet.
-Drizzle the olive oil over the Brussels sprouts and toss to coatSprinkle with salt and pepper to taste.
-Roast the Brussels sprouts in the preheated oven for 20-25 minutes, or until tender and lightly browned.
-Serve hot.

*Quinoa and Vegetable Salad*
Ingredients:

1 cup quinoa, rinsed and drained
2 cups water
1 red bell pepper, diced
1 yellow bell pepper, diced
1 cucumber, diced
1/4 cup chopped fresh parsley
1/4 cup chopped fresh mint
2 tbsp lemon juice
1 tbsp olive oil
Salt and pepper to taste

Instructions:
-In a medium saucepan, bring the quinoa and water to a boil.
-Reduce the heat to low and simmer, covered, for 15-20 minutes or until the quinoa is tender and the water is absorbed.
-In a large bowl, combine the cooked quinoa, diced red bell pepper, diced yellow bell pepper, diced cucumber, chopped fresh parsley, and chopped fresh mint.
-In a small bowl, whisk together the lemon juice, olive oil, salt, and pepper.
-Pour the dressing over the quinoa and vegetable mixture and toss to coat.

-Serve chilled.

*Steamed Broccoli*
Ingredients:
1 pound broccoli, cut into florets
Salt and pepper to taste

Instructions:
-Fill a large pot with an inch of water and bring to a boil.
-Place a steamer basket in the pot.
-Add the broccoli florets to the steamer basket and sprinkle with salt and pepper.
-Cover the pot and steam the broccoli for 5-7 minutes or until tender.
-Serve hot.

*Mashed Cauliflower*
Ingredients:
1 head cauliflower, cut into florets
1/4 cup low-fat milk
1 tbsp unsalted butter
Salt and pepper to taste

Instructions:

-Steam the cauliflower florets in a steamer basket for 8-10 minutes or until tender.
-Drain the cauliflower and transfer it to a food processor.
-Add the low-fat milk, unsalted butter, salt, and pepper to the food processor.
-Process the cauliflower until smooth and creamy.
-Serve hot.


*Roasted Sweet Potatoes*
Ingredients:
2 large sweet potatoes, peeled and diced
1 tbsp olive oil
Salt and pepper to taste

Instructions:
-Preheat the oven to 400°F (200°C).
-Place the diced sweet potatoes on a baking sheet.
-Drizzle the olive oil over the sweet potatoes and toss to coat.
-Sprinkle with salt and pepper to taste.
-Roast the sweet potatoes in the preheated oven for 20-25 minutes, or until tender and lightly browned.

Serve hot.

*Grilled Asparagus*
Ingredients:
1 lb. asparagus spears, trimmed
1 tbsp. olive oil
Salt and pepper to taste

Instructions:
-Preheat a grill or grill pan to medium-high heat.
-Toss the asparagus spears in the olive oil and season with salt and pepper.
-Grill the asparagus for 3-4 minutes per side, or until lightly charred and tender.
-Serve immediately.
Prep time: 10 minutes

*Roasted Brussels Sprouts with Balsamic Glaze*
Ingredients:
1 lb. Brussels sprouts, trimmed and halved
2 tbsp. olive oil
Salt and pepper to taste
1/4 cup balsamic vinegar
1 tbsp. honey

Instructions:
-Preheat the oven to 400°F (200°C).
-In a large bowl, toss the Brussels sprouts with the olive oil, salt, and pepper.
-Spread the Brussels sprouts out in a single layer on a baking sheet.
-Roast the Brussels sprouts for 20-25 minutes or until tender and lightly browned.
-In a small saucepan, whisk together the balsamic vinegar and honey.
-Bring the mixture to a boil and simmer for 5-7 minutes or until thickened.
-Drizzle the balsamic glaze over the roasted Brussels sprouts and serve.
Prep time: 15 minutes

:


*Garlic and Herb Roasted Cauliflower*
Ingredients:
1 head cauliflower, cut into florets
2 tbsp olive oil
2 cloves garlic, minced
1 tsp dried thyme
Salt and pepper to taste

Instructions:

-Preheat the oven to 400°F (200°C).

-In a large bowl, toss the cauliflower florets with olive oil, minced garlic, dried thyme, salt, and pepper.

-Spread the cauliflower on a baking sheet in a single layer.

-Roast in the oven for 20-25 minutes or until the cauliflower is golden brown and tender.

-Serve hot.

## *Balsamic Roasted Carrots*

Ingredients:

1 lb carrots, peeled and sliced

2 tbsp olive oil

2 tbsp balsamic vinegar

1 tsp honey

1 tsp dried rosemary

Salt and pepper to taste

Instructions:

-Preheat the oven to 400°F (200°C).

-In a large bowl, whisk together the olive oil, balsamic vinegar, honey, dried rosemary, salt, and pepper.

-Add the sliced carrots to the bowl and toss to coat.
-Spread the carrots on a baking sheet in a single layer.
-Roast in the oven for 20-25 minutes or until the carrots are tender.
-Serve hot.


*Sauteed Garlic Green Beans*
Ingredients:
1 lb green beans, trimmed
2 tbsp olive oil
3 cloves garlic, minced
Salt and pepper to taste

Instructions:
-In a large skillet, heat the olive oil over medium heat.
-Add the minced garlic to the skillet and cook until fragrant, stirring occasionally.
-Add the trimmed green beans to the skillet and toss to coat with the garlic and oil.
-Season with salt and pepper to taste.
-Cover the skillet and cook the green beans for 5-7 minutes or until tender.

Serve hot.


## *Cucumber Mint Water*
Ingredients:
1 cucumber, sliced
10-12 fresh mint leaves
8 cups water
Ice
Instructions:
-In a large pitcher, combine the sliced cucumber, mint leaves, and water.
-Stir well and refrigerate for at least 1 hour.
-Serve over ice.


## *Ginger and Lemon Tea*
Ingredients:
1 inch piece of fresh ginger, peeled and grated
1 lemon, juiced
4 cups water
Honey (optional)
Instructions:
-In a large pot, bring the water to a boil.
-Add the grated ginger to the pot and simmer for 10 minutes.
-Strain the ginger and discard.
-Stir in the lemon juice and honey (if desired).

-Serve hot.

*Pineapple and Turmeric Smoothie*
Ingredients:
1 cup fresh or frozen pineapple chunks
1 banana, peeled
1 tsp turmeric
1 cup unsweetened almond milk
1/4 tsp black pepper
Instructions:
-In a blender, combine the pineapple chunks, banana, turmeric, almond milk, and black pepper.
-Blend until smooth.
-Serve cold.

*Apple Cider Vinegar and Honey Drink*
Ingredients:
2 tbsp apple cider vinegar
1 tbsp honey
1 cup water
Ice
Instructions:
-In a glass, combine the apple cider vinegar, honey, and water.
-Stir well.

-Serve over ice.

*Green Tea with Lemon and Mint*
Ingredients:
2 green tea bags
4 cups water
1 lemon, sliced
10-12 fresh mint leaves
Instructions:
-In a large pot, bring the water to a boil.
-Add the green tea bags and steep for 3-4 minutes.
-Remove the tea bags and stir in the lemon slices and mint leaves.
-Let the tea cool to room temperature.
-Serve over ice.

*Blueberry and Spinach Smoothie*
Ingredients:
1 cup fresh or frozen blueberries
1 cup fresh spinach leaves
1 banana, peeled
1/2 cup unsweetened almond milk
Instructions:
-In a blender, combine the blueberries, spinach leaves, banana, and almond milk.

-Blend until smooth.
-Serve cold.


### Beet and Carrot Juice

Ingredients:

2 beets, peeled and chopped

4 carrots, peeled and chopped

1 apple, cored and chopped

1 inch piece of ginger, peeled and grated

Instructions:

-In a juicer, process the beets, carrots, apple, and ginger.

-Stir well.

-Serve cold.


### Mango Lassi

Ingredients:

1 cup plain low-fat yogurt

1 cup chopped fresh mango

1/2 cup unsweetened almond milk

1 tsp honey (optional)

Instructions:

-In a blender, combine the yogurt, chopped mango, almond milk, and honey (if desired).

-Blend until smooth.
-Serve cold.

*Pineapple Ginger Smoothie*
Ingredients:
1 cup frozen pineapple chunks
1-inch piece of fresh ginger root, peeled and sliced
1 banana
1 cup coconut water
Ice cubes
Instructions:
-In a blender, add the frozen pineapple chunks, sliced ginger root, banana, and coconut water.
-Blend until smooth.
-Add ice cubes to glasses and pour in the smoothie.
-Serve cold.

*Raspberry Lime Sparkling Water*
Ingredients:
1/2 cup fresh raspberries
2 limes, sliced
8 cups sparkling water
Ice cubes
Instructions:

-In a large pitcher, add the fresh raspberries and sliced limes to the sparkling water.
-Stir to combine, then chill in the refrigerator for at least 1 hour.
-Add ice cubes to glasses and pour in the raspberry lime sparkling water.
-Serve cold.

*Green Tea*
Ingredients:
2 green tea bags
4 cups water
Honey (optional)
Instructions:
-In a small pot, bring the water to a boil.
-Remove from heat and add the green tea bags.
-Steep the tea for 3-5 minutes.
-Remove the tea bags and add honey if desired.
-Serve hot.

*Beet and Carrot Juice*
Ingredients:
2 beets, peeled and chopped
4 carrots, peeled and chopped
1/2 lemon, juiced
2 cups water

Instructions:

-In a juicer, add the chopped beets and carrots.

-Juice the vegetables.

-Pour the juice into a large pitcher and add the lemon juice and water.

-Stir to combine.

-Serve chilled.

### Watermelon Agua Fresca

Ingredients:

4 cups watermelon, cubed

2 cups water

1/4 cup lime juice

1 tablespoon honey (optional)

Instructions:

-In a blender, add the cubed watermelon and water.

-Blend until smooth.

-Pour the mixture into a large pitcher and add the lime juice and honey (if using).

-Stir to combine.

-Serve chilled.

### Beet and Carrot Juice

Ingredients:

2 beets, peeled and chopped

2 carrots, peeled and chopped
1 apple, cored and chopped
1 inch piece of ginger, grated
Instructions:
-Add the chopped beets, carrots, apple, and grated ginger to a juicer.
-Process the ingredients until smooth.
-Pour the juice into a glass.
-Serve immediately.

*Turmeric Milk*
Ingredients:
2 cups milk
1 tsp ground turmeric
1/2 tsp ground cinnamon
1/2 tsp ground ginger
1 tbsp honey
Instructions:
-In a saucepan, heat the milk over medium heat.
-Add the ground turmeric, cinnamon, and ginger to the milk and whisk to combine.
-Simmer for 10-15 minutes, stirring occasionally.
-Add the honey and whisk to combine.
-Serve hot.

*Berry Smoothie*
Ingredients:
1 cup mixed berries (blueberries, raspberries, strawberries)
1 banana, peeled
1/2 cup low-fat yogurt
1/2 cup almond milk
1 tbsp honey
Instructions:
-Add the mixed berries, banana, low-fat yogurt, almond milk, and honey to a blender.
-Blend until smooth.
-Pour the smoothie into a glass.
-Serve cold.


*Pineapple Cucumber Juice*
Ingredients:
1 cup chopped pineapple
1 cucumber, chopped
1 lemon, juiced
1 tsp honey
Instructions:
-Add the chopped pineapple and cucumber to a juicer.
-Process the ingredients until smooth.

-Pour the juice into a glass.
-Add the lemon juice and honey to taste.
-Serve immediately.

*Iced Green Tea*
Ingredients:
4 green tea bags
8 cups water
1 lemon, sliced
1 tsp honey
Instructions:
-Boil 8 cups of water in a pot.
-Remove the pot from heat and add the green tea bags.
-Let the tea steep for 5-7 minutes.
-Remove the tea bags and let the tea cool to room temperature.
-Add the sliced lemon and honey to the tea.
-Refrigerate the iced tea for at least an hourbefore serving.
-Serve cold.

# Desserts And Treats

*Baked Apples with Cinnamon*
Ingredients:
4 apples, cored
2 tbsp honey
1 tsp cinnamon
1/4 cup chopped walnuts
Instructions:
-Preheat the oven to 375°F (190°C).
-In a small bowl, mix the honey and cinnamon.
-Brush the honey mixture over the cored apples.
-Place the apples in a baking dish and sprinkle with chopped walnuts.
-Bake for 25-30 minutes, or until the apples are soft and the topping is golden brown.
-Serve warm.

*Chocolate Banana Pudding*
Ingredients:
2 ripe bananas, mashed
1/4 cup cocoa powder
1/4 cup honey
1 tsp vanilla extract

1/4 cup almond milk

Instructions:

-In a large bowl, mix the mashed bananas, cocoa powder, honey, and vanilla extract.

-Add the almond milk and stir until smooth.

-Spoon the mixture into small dessert cups.

-Refrigerate for at least an hour before serving.

-Serve chilled.

## *Berry Crumble*

Ingredients:

2 cups mixed berries (blueberries, raspberries, strawberries)

1/2 cup rolled oats

1/4 cup almond flour

1/4 cup chopped walnuts

1/4 cup honey

1/4 cup coconut oil, melted

Instructions:

-Preheat the oven to 375°F (190°C).

-In a large bowl, mix the mixed berries, rolled oats, almond flour, chopped walnuts, and honey.

-Drizzle the melted coconut oil over the mixture and stir to combine.

-Spoon the mixture into a baking dish.
-Bake for 25-30 minutes, or until the topping is golden brown and the fruit is bubbling.
-Serve warm.


*Avocado Chocolate Mousse*
Ingredients:
2 ripe avocados, peeled and pitted
1/2 cup cocoa powder
1/2 cup honey
1 tsp vanilla extract
Instructions:
-In a blender, blend the avocados, cocoa powder, honey, and vanilla extract until smooth.
-Spoon the mixture into small dessert cups.
-Refrigerate for at least an hour before serving.
-Serve chilled.


*Baked Pears with Honey and Yogurt*
Ingredients:
4 pears, halved and cored
2 tbsp honey
1/2 cup low-fat yogurt
Instructions:
-Preheat the oven to 375°F (190°C).

-Place the pear halves in a baking dish.
-Drizzle the honey over the pears.
-Bake for 25-30 minutes, or until the pears are soft and the honey is golden brown.
-Serve with a dollop of low-fat yogurt on top.

*Berry Sorbet*
Ingredients:
2 cups mixed berries (blueberries, raspberries, strawberries)
1/4 cup honey
1/4 cup water
Instructions:
-In a blender, blend the mixed berries, honey, and water until smooth.
-Pour the mixture into a shallow dish.
-Freeze for 2 hours, stirring every 30 minutes, until the sorbet is firm.
-Serve chilled.

*Chocolate Banana Bites*
Ingredients:
2 bananas, sliced
1/2 cup dark chocolate chips
1 tsp coconut oil

Instructions:
-Line a baking sheet with parchment paper.
-Place the sliced bananas on the baking sheet.
-Melt the dark chocolate chips and coconut oil in a microwave-safe bowl.
-Drizzle the melted chocolate over the banana slices.
-Freeze the chocolate banana bites for at least an hour before serving.
-Serve cold.

*Berry Sorbet*
Ingredients:
2 cups mixed berries (blueberries, raspberries, strawberries)
1/4 cup honey
1/4 cup water
Instructions:
-Add the mixed berries, honey, and water to a blender.
-Blend until smooth.
-Pour the mixture into a freezer-safe container.
-Freeze the berry sorbet for at least 3 hours, stirring every hour to prevent crystallization.
-Serve cold.

*Coconut Chia Pudding*

Ingredients:

1/2 cup chia seeds

1 1/2 cups coconut milk

1 tsp vanilla extract

1 tbsp honey

Shredded coconut, for topping

Instructions:

-In a large bowl, whisk together the chia seeds, coconut milk, vanilla extract, and honey.

-Cover the bowl and refrigerate for at least 2 hours, or overnight.

-Stir the chia pudding before serving.

-Top with shredded coconut.

-Serve cold.


*Roasted Pear with Yogurt*

Ingredients:

2 pears, halved and cored

1 tsp cinnamon

2 tbsp honey

1/2 cup low-fat yogurt

Instructions:

-Preheat the oven to 375°F.

-Place the pear halves in a baking dish.

-Sprinkle cinnamon over the pears.

-Drizzle honey over the pears.

-Roast the pears for 20-25 minutes, until soft and caramelized.

-Serve the roasted pears with a dollop of low-fat yogurt.

*Almond Butter Cookies*

Ingredients:

1 cup almond butter

1/2 cup honey

1 egg

1 tsp vanilla extract

Instructions:

-Preheat the oven to 350°F.

-In a large bowl, mix together the almond butter, honey, egg, and vanilla extract.

-Form the cookie dough into balls and place them on a baking sheet lined with parchment paper.

-Flatten the cookie dough balls with a fork.

-Bake the almond butter cookies for 10-12 minutes.

-Let the cookies cool before serving.

<u>*Frozen Grapes*</u>
Ingredients:
2 cups grapes
Instructions:
-Wash and dry the grapes.
-Freeze the grapes for at least an hour before serving.
-Serve cold.

<u>*Banana Oat Bars:*</u>
Ingredients:
2 ripe bananas, mashed
1 1/2 cups rolled oats
1/4 cup almond flour
1/4 cup honey
1/4 cup coconut oil, melted
1 tsp vanilla extract
1/2 tsp ground cinnamon
1/4 tsp salt
Optional: chopped nuts, chocolate chips, or dried fruit for toppings
Instructions:
-Preheat the oven to 350°F (175°C) and grease an 8x8 inch baking dish.
-In a large mixing bowl, combine the mashed bananas, rolled oats, almond flour, honey,

melted coconut oil, vanilla extract, ground cinnamon, and salt.
-Mix well until fully combined.
-Pour the mixture into the greased baking dish and spread it out evenly.
-Optional: sprinkle chopped nuts, chocolate chips, or dried fruit on top of the mixture.
-Bake for 25-30 minutes, or until the edges are golden brown and the center is set.
-Remove from the oven and let cool for 10 minutes before cutting into squares.
Serve and enjoy!
Prep time: 10 minutes
Cook time: 25-30 minutes
Total time: 35-40 minutes

*Apple Nachos*
Ingredients:
1 apple, sliced
1 tbsp almond butter
1 tbsp unsweetened shredded coconut
1 tbsp chopped walnuts
1 tbsp dark chocolate chips
Instructions:
-Arrange the apple slices on a plate.
Drizzle with almond butter.

-Sprinkle with shredded coconut, chopped walnuts, and dark chocolate chips.
Serve immediately.
Prep time: 5 minutes


*Banana Ice Cream*
Ingredients:
2 ripe bananas, sliced and frozen
1 tbsp almond butter
1 tbsp unsweetened shredded coconut
1 tbsp chopped walnuts
Instructions:
-Add the frozen banana slices to a food processor.
-Blend until smooth and creamy.
-Serve topped with almond butter, shredded coconut, and chopped walnuts.
Prep time: 10 minutes


*Dark Chocolate Dipped Strawberries*
Ingredients:
1 cup fresh strawberries
1/4 cup dark chocolate chips
1 tsp coconut oil
Instructions:
-Line a baking sheet with parchment paper.

-In a microwave-safe bowl, melt the dark chocolate chips and coconut oil together in 30-second intervals, stirring in between, until fully melted.
-Dip each strawberry in the melted chocolate and place on the lined baking sheet.
-Refrigerate until the chocolate is set.
Serve and enjoy.
Prep time: 20 minutes


*Yogurt Parfait*
Ingredients:
1 cup plain Greek yogurt
1/2 cup mixed berries
2 tbsp unsweetened granola
1 tbsp chopped almonds
Instructions:
-In a small glass, layer the Greek yogurt, mixed berries, and granola.
-Top with chopped almonds.
-Serve and enjoy.
Prep time: 10 minutes


*Cinnamon Roasted Almonds*
Ingredients:
1 cup raw almonds

1 tbsp coconut oil
1 tbsp maple syrup
1 tsp cinnamon
Instructions:
-Preheat the oven to 350°F.
-In a bowl, mix together the almonds, coconut oil, maple syrup, and cinnamon.
-Spread the almond mixture on a baking sheet.
-Bake for 10-15 minutes, or until the almonds are lightly browned.
-Serve and enjoy.
Prep time: 20 minutes


*Apple Cinnamon Oatmeal Cookies*
Ingredients:
2 cups rolled oats
1 cup unsweetened applesauce
1/4 cup honey
1 tsp vanilla extract
1 tsp cinnamon
1/2 tsp baking powder
Pinch of salt
Instructions:
-Preheat oven to 350°F (175°C).

-In a large bowl, combine all ingredients and mix well.
-Scoop the mixture onto a baking sheet lined with parchment paper.
-Bake for 10-12 minutes, or until lightly golden.
-Allow to cool before serving.
Prep time: 15 minutes

*Chocolate Avocado Pudding*
Ingredients:
2 ripe avocados
1/2 cup unsweetened cocoa powder
1/2 cup maple syrup
1 tsp vanilla extract
Pinch of salt
Instructions:
-In a food processor, blend all ingredients until smooth and creamy.
-Spoon the mixture into serving dishes.
-Refrigerate for at least 30 minutes before serving.
Prep time: 10 minutes

*Baked Sweet Potato Chips*
Ingredients:
2 sweet potatoes, thinly sliced

2 tbsp olive oil

1 tsp paprika

1/2 tsp garlic powder

Pinch of salt

Instructions:

-Preheat oven to 375°F (190°C).

-In a bowl, toss the sweet potato slices with olive oil, paprika, garlic powder, and salt.

-Spread the slices in a single layer on a baking sheet lined with parchment paper.

-Bake for 15-20 minutes, or until crispy and golden.

-Allow to cool before serving.

Prep time: 10 minutes

## _Blueberry Banana Ice Cream_

Ingredients:

2 frozen bananas, sliced

1/2 cup frozen blueberries

1/4 cup unsweetened almond milk

Instructions:

-In a blender or food processor, blend all ingredients until smooth and creamy.

Serve immediately, or freeze for later use.

Prep time: 5 minutes

*<u>Dark Chocolate Almond Butter Cups</u>*
Ingredients:
1/2 cup dark chocolate chips
1/4 cup almond butter
Instructions:
-Line a muffin tin with 6 paper liners.
-In a microwave-safe bowl, melt the dark chocolate chips in 30-second intervals, stirring in between, until fully melted.
-Spoon about 1 tablespoon of the melted chocolate into each paper liner, spreading it up the sides.
-Spoon about 1 teaspoon of almond butter on top of the melted chocolate in each liner.
-Top with another tablespoon of melted chocolate, spreading it over the almond butter to completely cover.
-Repeat with the remaining liners.
-Refrigerate for at least 30 minutes, or until the chocolate has hardened.
-Remove the paper liners from the almond butter cups.
-Serve and enjoy!
Prep time: 10 minutes
Total time: 40 minutes

# Conclusion

In conclusion, Nourishing Recipes For A Healthy Gallbladder: Delicious Meals for Optimal Digestion is an excellent resource for anyone seeking to improve their digestive health and overall well-being. This cookbook is a comprehensive guide that provides a wealth of information about the gallbladder and its crucial role in the digestive system.

The recipes contained in this cookbook are not only delicious but also nutrient-dense and carefully crafted to support gallbladder health. Each recipe has been designed to include specific ingredients that are beneficial for digestion, such as healthy fats, fiber, and antioxidants.

Moreover, this cookbook provides a variety of recipes that cater to different dietary requirements, including vegetarian, gluten-free, and dairy-free options. This ensures that everyone can benefit from the recipes in this cookbook, regardless of their dietary restrictions.

Furthermore, the cookbook includes practical tips on how to incorporate healthy eating habits into daily life, such as meal planning and preparation. These tips can help individuals stay on track and maintain a healthy diet that supports optimal digestion.

Overall, Nourishing Recipes For A Healthy Gallbladder: Delicious Meals for Optimal Digestion is a valuable resource for anyone seeking to improve their digestive health and overall well-being. By following the recipes and tips in this cookbook, individuals can nourish their bodies and support their gallbladder health.